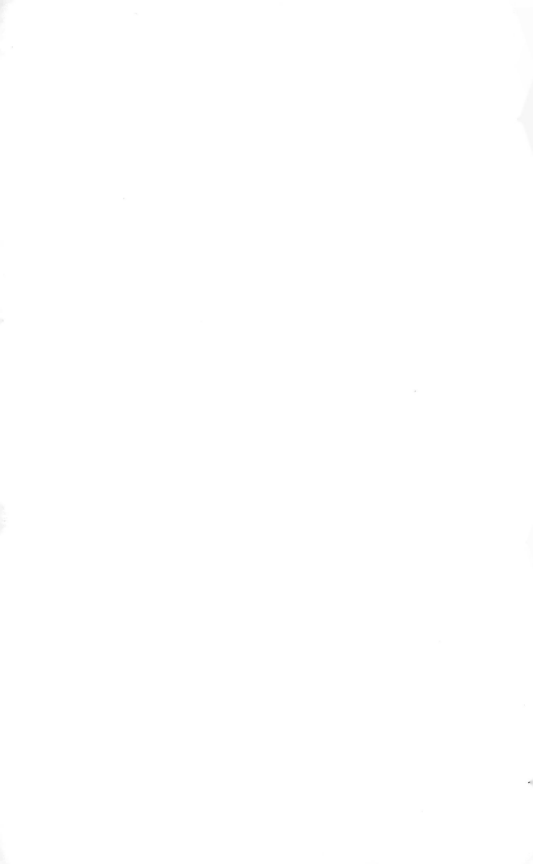

Vibrant
New Mediterranean
Diet Cookbook

Quick and Delicious Diner Recipes to Burn Fat

Jude Barnes

Table of Contents

Fig and Prosciutto Pita Bread Pizza

Preparation Time:

5 minutes

Cooking Time:

20 minutes

Servings: 6

Ingredients:

- 4 pita breads
- 8 figs, quartered
- 8 slices prosciutto
- 8 ounces mozzarella, crumbled

Directions:

1. Set the pita bread on a baking plate.
2. Top with crumbled cheese then figs and prosciutto.
3. Bake at 350°F for 8 minutes.
4. Serve the pizza right away.

Nutrition:

- Calories: 445
- Fat: 13.7 g
- Carbs: 41.5 g
- Protein: 39.0 g

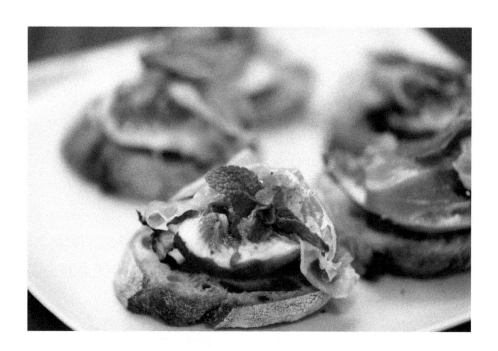

Spaghetti in Clam Sauce

Preparation Time:

5 minutes

Cooking Time:

45 minutes

Servings: 4

Ingredients:

- 8 ounces spaghetti
- 2 tablespoons olive oil
- 2 garlic cloves, minced
- 2 tomatoes, peeled and diced
- 1 cup cherry tomatoes, halved
- 1-pound fresh clams, cleaned and rinsed
- 2 tablespoons white wine
- 1 teaspoon sherry vinegar

Directions:

1. Heat the oil and add the garlicups
2. Cook until fragrant, then attach the tomatoes, wine, and vinegar.
3. Boil and cook, then stir in the clams and continue cooking for 10 more minutes.
4. Boil water with a pinch of salt and add the spaghetti.

5. Cook for 8 minutes just until al dente. Drain well and mix with the clam sauce.

6. Serve the dish right away.

Nutrition:

- Calories: 305
- Fat: 8.8 g
- Carbs: 48.3 g
- Protein: 8.1 g

Creamy Fish Gratin

Preparation Time:

5 minutes

Cooking Time:

1 hour

Servings: 6

Ingredients:

- 1 cup heavy cream
- 2 salmon fillets, cubed
- 2 cod fillets, cubed
- 2 sea bass fillets, cubed
- 1 celery stalk, sliced
- Salt and pepper to taste
- 1/2 cup grated Parmesan
- 1/2 cup feta cheese, crumbled

Directions:

1. Combine the cream with the fish fillets and celery in a deep-dish baking pan.
2. Add salt and pepper to taste, then top with the Parmesan and feta cheese.
3. Cook in the oven for 20 minutes.
4. Serve the gratin right away.

Nutrition:

- Calories: 300
- Fat: 16.1 g
- Carbs: 1.3
- Protein: 36.9 g

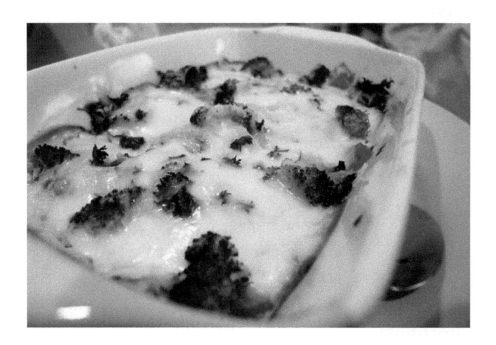

Broccoli Pesto Spaghetti

Preparation Time:

5 minutes

Cooking Time:

35 minutes

Servings: 4

Ingredients:

- 8 ounces spaghetti
- 1-pound broccoli, cut into florets
- 2 tablespoons olive oil
- 4 garlic cloves, chopped
- 4 basil leaves
- 2 tablespoons blanched almonds
- 1 lemon, juiced
- Salt and pepper to taste

Directions:

1. For the pesto, combine the broccoli, oil, garlic, basil, lemon juice, and almonds in a blender and pulse until well mixed and smooth.
2. Cook the pasta in salty water for 8 minutes or until al dente.
3. Drain well.
4. Mix the warm spaghetti with the broccoli pesto and serve right away.

Nutrition:

- Calories: 284
- Fat: 10.2 g
- Carbs: 40.2 g
- Protein: 10.4 g

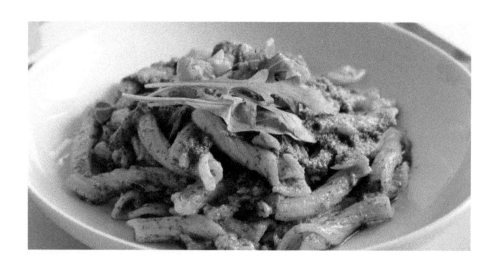

Spaghetti all 'Olio

Preparation Time:

5 minutes

Cooking Time:

30 minutes

Servings: 4

Ingredients:

- 8 ounces spaghetti
- 3 tablespoons olive oil
- 4 garlic cloves, minced
- 2 red peppers, sliced
- 1 tablespoon lemon juice
- Salt and pepper to taste
- 1/2 cup grated parmesan cheese

Directions:

1. Heat the oil and attach the garlicups
2. Cook, then whip in the red peppers and cook for 1 more minute on low heat, making sure to only infuse them, not to burn or fry them.
3. Add the lemon juice and remove off heat.

4. Cook the pasta with salty water for 8 minutes or as stated on the package, just until they become al dente.

5. Drain the spaghetti well and mix them with the garlic and pepper oil.

6. Serve right away.

Nutrition:

- Calories: 268
- Fat: 11.9 g
- Carbs: 34.1 g
- Protein: 7.1 g

Quick Tomato Spaghetti

Preparation Time:

5 minutes

Cooking Time:

15 minutes

Servings: 4

Ingredients:

- 8 ounces spaghetti
- 3 tablespoons olive oil
- 4 garlic cloves, sliced
- 1 jalapeno, sliced
- 2 cups cherry tomatoes
- Salt and pepper to taste
- 1 teaspoon balsamic vinegar
- 1/2 cup grated Parmesan

Directions:

1. Heat a large pot of water on medium flame.
2. Add a pinch of salt and bring to a boil, then add the pasta.
3. Cook until al dente.
4. While the pasta cooks, heat the oil in a skillet and add the garlic and jalapeno.

5. Cook, then blend in the tomatoes, as well as salt and pepper.

6. Cook for 5-7 minutes until the tomatoes' skins burst.

7. Add the vinegar and remove off heat.

8. Unload the pasta well and merge it with the tomato sauce.

9. Sprinkle with cheese and serve right away.

Nutrition:

- Calories: 298
- Fat: 13.5 g
- Carbs: 36.0 g

  Protein: 9.7 g

Creamy Chicken Soup

Preparation Time:

10 minutes

Cooking Time:

1 hour

Servings: 8

Ingredients:

- 2 cups eggplant, cubed
- Salt and black pepper to the taste
- 1/4 cup olive oil
- 1 yellow onion, chopped
- 2 tablespoons garlic, minced
- 1 red bell pepper, chopped
- 2 tablespoons hot paprika
- 1/4 cup parsley, chopped
- 1 1/2 tablespoons oregano, chopped
- 4 cups chicken stock
- 1 pound chicken breast, skinless, boneless, and cubed
- 1 cup half and half
- 2 egg yolks
- 1/4 cup lime juice

Directions:

1. Heat up a pot with the oil over medium heat, add the chicken, garlic, and onion, and brown for 10 minutes.

2. Attach the bell pepper and merge the rest of the ingredients except the half and half, egg, yolks, and the lime juice, bring to a simmer and cook over medium heat for 40 minutes.

3. Merge the egg yolks with the remaining ingredients with 1 cup of soup, whisk well, and pour into the pot.

4. Whisk the soup, cook for 5 minutes more, divide into bowls, and serve.

Nutrition:

- Calories: 312
- Fat: 17.4 g
- Fiber: 5.6 g
- Carbs: 20.2 g
- Protein: 15.3 g

Chili Oregano Baked Cheese

Preparation Time:

5 minutes

Cooking Time:

35 minutes

Servings: 4

Ingredients:

- 8 ounces feta cheese
- 4 ounces mozzarella, crumbled
- 1 chili pepper, sliced
- 1 teaspoon dried oregano
- 2 tablespoons olive oil

Directions:

1. Place the feta cheese in a small deep-dish baking pan.
2. Top with the mozzarella, then season with pepper slices and oregano.
3. Shield the pan with aluminum foil and bake in the preheated oven.
4. Serve the cheese right away.

Nutrition:

- Calories: 292
- Fat: 24.2 g
- Carbs: 3.7 g
- Protein: 16.2 g

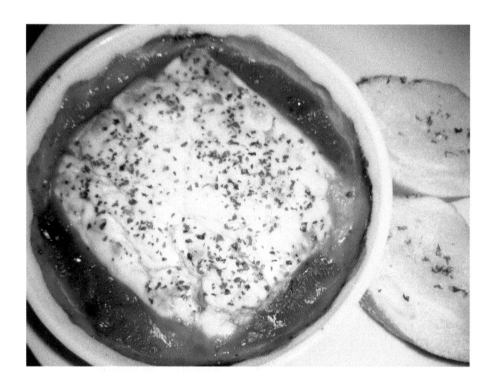

Barley and Chicken Soup

Preparation Time:

10 minutes

Cooking Time:

50 minutes

Servings: 6

Ingredients:

- 1 pound chicken breasts, skinless, boneless, and cubed
- 1 tablespoon olive oil
- Salt and black pepper to the taste
- 2 celery stalks, chopped
- 2 carrots, chopped
- 1 red onion, chopped
- 6 cups chicken stock
- 1/2 cup parsley, chopped
- 1/2 cup barley
- 1 teaspoon lime juice

Directions:

1. Heat up a pot with the oil over medium-high heat, add the chicken, season with salt and pepper, and cook for 8 minutes until brown.
2. Add the onion, carrots, and celery, stir and cook for 3 minutes more.

3. Attach the rest of the ingredients except the parsley, bring to a boil and simmer over medium heat for 40 minutes.

4. Add the parsley, stir, divide the soup into bowls, and serve.

Nutrition:

- Calories: 311
- Fat: 8.4 g
- Fiber: 8.3 g
- Carbs: 17.4 g
- Protein: 22.3 g

Crispy Italian Chicken

Preparation Time:

5 minutes

Cooking Time:

40 minutes

Servings: 4

Ingredients:

- 4 chicken legs
- 1 teaspoon dried basil
- 1 teaspoon dried oregano
- Salt and pepper to taste
- 3 tablespoons olive oil
- 1 tablespoon balsamic vinegar

Directions:

1. Season the chicken with salt, pepper, basil, and oregano.
2. Heat the oil and attach the chicken to the hot oil.
3. Cook on each side until golden, then cover the skillet with a weight another skillet or a very heavy lid is recommended.

4. Place over medium heat and cook for 10 minutes on one side, then flip the chicken repeatedly, cooking for another 10 minutes until crispy.

5. Serve the chicken right away.

Nutrition:

- Calories: 262
- Fat: 13.9 g
- Carbs: 0.3 g
- Protein: 32.6 g

Sea Bass in a Pocket

Preparation Time:

5 minutes

Cooking Time:

40 minutes

Servings: 4

Ingredients:

- 4 sea bass fillets
- 4 garlic cloves, sliced
- 1 celery stalk, sliced
- 1 zucchini, sliced
- 1 cup cherry tomatoes, halved
- 1 shallot, sliced
- 1 teaspoon dried oregano
- Salt and pepper to taste

Directions:

1. Mix the garlic, celery, zucchini, tomatoes, shallot, and oregano in a bowl.
2. Add salt and pepper to taste.
3. Take 4 sheets of baking paper and arrange them on your working surface. Spoon the vegetable mixture in the center of each sheet.

4. Top with a fish fillet, then wrap the paper well so it resembles a pocket.

5. Place the wrapped fish in a baking tray and cook in the preheated oven at 350°F for 15 minutes.

6. Serve the fish warm and fresh.

Nutrition:

- Calories: 149
- Fat: 2.8 g
- Carbs: 5.2 g
- Protein: 25.2 g

Chicken and Chorizo Casserole

Preparation Time:

5 minutes

Cooking Time:

1 hour

Servings: 6

Ingredients:

- 6 chicken thighs
- 4 chorizo links, sliced
- 2 tablespoons olive oil
- 1 cup tomato juice
- 2 tablespoons tomato paste
- 1 bay leaf
- 1 teaspoon dried thyme
- Salt and pepper to taste

Directions:

1. Heat the oil and attach the chicken.
2. Cook on all sides until golden then transfer the chicken to a deep-dish baking pan.
3. Attach the rest of the ingredients and pour them with salt and pepper.
4. Cook in the preheated oven.
5. Serve the casserole right away.

Nutrition:

- Calories: 424
- Fat: 27.5 g
- Carbs: 3.6 g
- Protein: 39.1 g

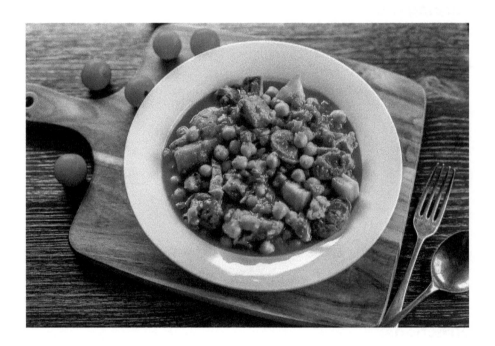

Lamb Stuffed Tomatoes with Herbs

Preparation Time:

5 minutes

Cooking Time:

1 hour

Servings: 6

Ingredients:

- 6 large tomatoes
- 1-pound ground lamb
- 1/4 cup white rice
- 2 shallots, chopped
- 2 garlic cloves, minced
- 1 tablespoon chopped dill
- 1 tablespoon chopped parsley
- 1 tablespoon chopped cilantro
- 1 teaspoon dried mint
- Salt and pepper to taste
- 1 tablespoon lemon juice
- 2 tablespoons olive oil
- 1 cup vegetable stock

Directions:

1. Mix the lamb, rice, shallots, garlic, dill, parsley, cilantro, and mint in a bowl.

2. Add salt and pepper to taste.

3. Remove the top of each tomato, then carefully remove the flesh, leaving the skins intact.

4. Chop the flesh finely and place it in a deep heavy saucepan.

5. Add the lemon juice, as well as salt and pepper to taste.

6. Stuff the tomatoes with the lamb mixture and place them all in the pan.

7. Drizzle with oil, then pour in the stock.

8. Cover with a lid and cook on low heat for 35 minutes.

9. Serve the tomatoes right away.

Nutrition:

- Calories: 248
- Fat: 10.7 g
- Carbs: 14.6 g
- Protein: 23.7 g

Creamy Spinach with Polenta and Poached Egg

Preparation Time:

5 minutes

Cooking Time:

40 minutes

Servings: 4

Ingredients:

For the Creamy Spinach:
- 2 tablespoons olive oil
- 2 garlic cloves, minced
- 1 red pepper, chopped
- 4 cups baby spinach
- 1/2 cup heavy cream
- 1 tablespoon all-purpose flour
- Salt and pepper to taste

For the Polenta:
- 1/2 cup polenta flour
- 1 1/2 cups water
- 1 tablespoon olive oil
- Salt and pepper to taste

For the Poached Eggs:

- 3 cups water
- 1 tablespoon white wine vinegar
- 4 eggs

Directions:

1. For the creamy spinach, heat the oil in a skillet and add the garlic and red pepper.
2. Cook, then attach the spinach and continue cooking for 5-7 minutes until the spinach is softened and most of the liquid has evaporated.
3. Mix the cream with the flour and pour it over the spinach.
4. Cook for 5 more minutes until thick and creamy.
5. For the polenta, heat the water with salt.
6. When boiled, stir in the oil and polenta flour.
7. Cook on low heat for 10 minutes.
8. For the poached eggs, bring the water, vinegar, and a pinch of salt to a boil in a saucepan.
9. To serve, spoon the polenta on the servings plates. Top with creamy spinach and finish with a poached egg.

Nutrition:

- Calories: 231
- Fat: 20.7 g
- Carbs: 5.7 g
- Protein: 7.3 g

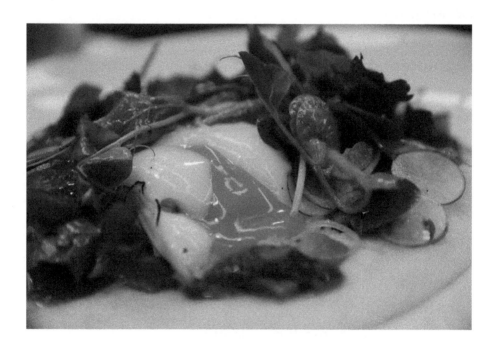

Grilled Vegetable Feta Tart

Preparation Time:

5 minutes

Cooking Time:

1 1/2 hours

Servings: 8

Ingredients:

For the Crust:

- 2 cups all-purpose flour
- 1 teaspoon instant yeast
- 1/2 teaspoon salt
- 1 cup water
- 2 tablespoons olive oil

For the Topping:

- 1 zucchini, sliced
- 2 tomatoes, sliced
- 1 shallot, sliced
- 1 teaspoon dried basil
- 1 teaspoon dried oregano
- 2 garlic cloves, minced
- 2 tablespoons tomato paste
- 4 ounces feta cheese, crumbled

Directions:

1. Merge all the ingredients in a bowl and mix well. Knead for a few minutes until elasticups

2. Let the dough rise, then roll it into a thin round of dough.

3. Place the dough on a baking tray.

4. Mix the garlic, basil, oregano, and tomato paste in a bowl.

5. Spread the mixture over the dough.

6. Heat a grill pan and place the zucchini and tomatoes on the grill. Cook for a few minutes on all sides until browned.

7. Top the tart with the vegetables and shallot, then sprinkle the cheese on top.

8. Bake in the oven for 25 minutes.

9. Serve the tart warm and fresh.

Nutrition:

- Calories: 198
- Fat: 7.0 g
- Carbs: 28.0 g
- Protein: 6.3 g

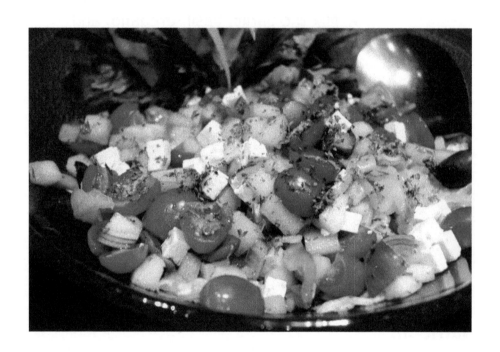

Yogurt Baked Eggplants

Preparation Time:

5 minutes

Cooking Time:

45 minutes

Servings: 4

Ingredients:

- 2 eggplants
- 4 garlic cloves, minced
- 1 teaspoon dried basil
- 2 tablespoons lemon juice
- Salt and pepper to taste
- 1 cup Greek yogurt
- 2 tablespoons chopped parsley

Directions:

1. Divide the eggplants in half and score the halves with a sharp knife.
2. Season the eggplants with salt and pepper, as well as the basil, then drizzle with lemon juice and place the eggplant halves on a baking tray.
3. Spread the garlic over the eggplants and bake in the preheated oven at 350°F for 20 minutes.

4. When done, place the eggplants on serving plates and top with yogurt and parsley.

5. Serve the eggplants right away.

Nutrition:

- Calories: 113
- Fat: 1.6 g
- Carbs: 19.4 g
- Protein: 8.1 g

Asparagus Baked Plaice

Preparation Time:

5 minutes

Cooking Time:

45 minutes

Servings: 4

Ingredients:

- 4 plaice fillets
- 2 cups cherry tomatoes
- 1 bunch asparagus, trimmed and halved
- 1/2 lemon, juiced
- 2 tablespoons olive oil
- Salt and pepper to taste

Directions:

1. Combine the tomatoes, asparagus, lemon juice, and oil in a deep-dish baking pan.
2. Season with salt and pepper.
3. Place the fillets on top and cook in the preheated oven at 350°F for 15 minutes.
4. Serve the plaice and the veggies warm and fresh.

41

Nutrition:

- Calories: 113
- Fat: 1.6 g
- Carbs: 19.4 g
- Protein: 8.1 g

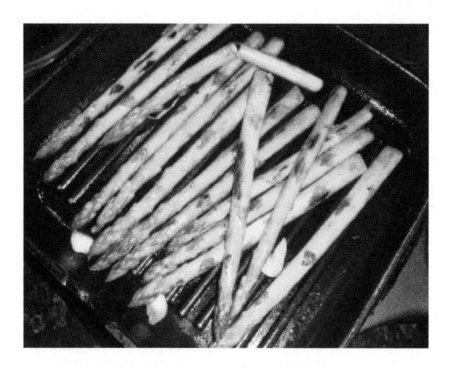

Vegetable Turkey Casserole

Preparation Time:

5 minutes

Cooking Time:

1 1/2 hours

Servings: 8

Ingredients:

- 3 tablespoons olive oil
- 2 pounds turkey breasts, cubed
- 1 sweet onion, chopped
- 3 carrots, sliced
- 2 celery stalks, sliced
- 2 garlic cloves, chopped
- 1/2 teaspoon cumin powder
- 1/2 teaspoon dried thyme
- 2 cans diced tomatoes
- 1 cup chicken stock
- 1 bay leaf
- Salt and pepper to taste

Directions:

1. Heat the oil and stir in the turkey.
2. Cook for 5 minutes until golden on all sides, then add the onion, carrot, celery, and garlicups.

3. Cook, then attach the rest of the ingredients.

4. Season with salt and pepper and cook in the preheated oven.

5. Serve the casserole warm and fresh.

Nutrition:

- Calories: 186
- Fat: 7.3 g
- Protein: 20.1 g

Mushroom Pilaf

Preparation Time:

5 minutes

Cooking Time:

50 minutes

Servings: 4

Ingredients:

- 2 tablespoons olive oil
- 1 shallot, chopped
- 2 garlic cloves, minced
- 1 pound button mushrooms
- 1 cup brown rice
- 2 cups chicken stock
- 1 bay leaf
- 1 thyme sprig
- Salt and pepper to taste

Directions:

1. Heat the oil and whip in the shallot and garlicups.
2. Cook until softened and fragrant.
3. Attach the mushrooms and rice and cook for 5 minutes.

4. Add the stock, bay leaf, and thyme, as well as salt and pepper, and continue cooking for 20 more minutes on low heat.

5. Serve the pilaf warm and fresh.

Nutrition:

- Calories: 265
- Fat: 8.9 g
- Carbs: 41.2 g
- Protein: 7.6 g

Summer Fish Stew

Preparation Time:

5 minutes

Cooking Time:

1 hour

Servings: 6

Ingredients:

- 3 tablespoons olive oil
- 4 garlic cloves, minced
- 1 red onion, chopped
- 1 celery stalk, sliced
- 2 red bell peppers, cored and diced
- 2 tablespoons tomato paste
- 2 cups cherry tomatoes
- 1 cup vegetable stock
- Salt and pepper to taste
- 4 cod fillets, cubed
- 4 sea bass fillets, cubed
- 2 tablespoons all-purpose flour

Directions:

1. Drizzle the fish with salt and pepper, then sprinkle it with flour.

2. Heat the oil in a skillet, then place the fish and cook it on all sides until golden brown.

3. It just must be golden brown, not cooked through just yet.

4. Remove the fish on a platter.

5. Add the garlic, onion, and celery in the same skillet as the fish was in and cook for 2 minutes until fragrant.

6. Whip in the remaining ingredients and season with salt and pepper.

7. Cook for 10 minutes on low heat, then add the fish and cook for another 10 minutes.

8. Serve the stew warm and fresh.

Nutrition:

- Calories: 318
- Fat: 10.1 g
- Carbs: 10.3 g
- Protein: 45.1 g

Italian Zucchini Meatballs

Preparation Time:

10 minutes

Cooking Time:

46 minutes

Servings: 6

Ingredients:

- For the Meatballs
- Turkey sausage, Italian, casings removed*, 16 oz., (2 Leans)
- Mozzarella cheese, low fat, 1 cup, (1 Lean)
- Parmesan cheese, low fat, 6 tbsp., (3 Condiments)
- Shredded zucchini, 1 cup (2 Greens)
- Salt, 3/4 tsp., (3 Condiments)
- Onion powder, 2 tsp. (4 Condiments)
- Minced garlic, fresh, 2 tsp. (2 Condiments)
- Italian seasoning, 1 tsp. (2 Condiments)
- Egg, 1, (1/3 Lean)
- For the Topping
- Marinara sauce, approved, 1 cup (4 Greens)
- Mozzarella cheese, low fat, 2/3 cup (2/3 Lean)

- Chopped fresh basil, 1/4 cup, (1/4 Condiment)

Directions:

1. Heat the oven to 400 degrees.
2. Apply cooking spray on the baking dish.
3. After shredding the zucchini, squeeze out the extra moisture from it through a clean cloth.
4. In a large bowl, mix all the ingredients to be used for meatballs.
5. Scoop out small meatballs using a scooper and put them on the baking sheet.
6. Cook for 20 to 26 min or till fully baked. Drain the oil.
7. Season with 2/3 cup cheese and marinara sauce.
8. Until cheese melts, bake for about 5 to 10 minutes extra.
9. Adorn it with fresh basil.

Nutrition:

Energy (calories): 110 kcal

Protein: 1.07 g Fat: 0.41 g Carbohydrates: 0.53 g

Meaty Taco Dip

Preparation Time:

10 minutes

Cooking Time:

35 minutes

Servings: 6

Ingredients:

- Turkey or lean ground beef, 95 to 97%, 1 1/2 lb.
- Tomato sauce, 1/2 cup
- Taco seasoning, 3 tbsp., divided
- Green chiles, diced, 4 oz.
- Greek yogurt, plain, 2%, 1 1/2 cups
- Softened cream cheese, low fat, and 6 oz.
- Cheddar cheese, low fat, shredded, 2 cups
- Shredded iceberg lettuce, 2 cups
- Tomatoes, chopped, 1/2 cup
- Jalapeno slices, 1 oz., from a jar
- Green onions, for garnish

Directions:

1. Crumble the ground beef and cook in a large pan. Remove the extra fat.

2. Put in tomato sauce, green chiles, and two tablespoon taco seasoning, stirring until combined.

3. Cook for 2 minutes. A 13 x 9-inch dish, spread the mixture of ground beef and let it come to room temperature.

4. Mix the soft cream cheese, Greek yogurt, and one tablespoon taco seasoning into a bowl till fully combined with a hand mixture. It should be spread over the ground beef.

5. On the top, scatter lettuce, cheese, and tomatoes.

6. Put on the sliced jalapenos and adorn with green onions. Equally divide into six portions. For up to three days can keep in the fridge.

Nutrition:

Energy (calories): 241 kcal Protein: 25.31 g Fat: 11.16 g Carbohydrates: 7.2 g

Jalapeno Popper Chicken Dip

Preparation Time:

10 minutes

Cooking Time:

30 minutes

Servings: 4

Ingredients:

- Shredded, skinless chicken breasts, boneless, cooked, 12 oz. (2 leans)
- Plain Greek yogurt, low fat, 3/4 cups, (1/2 lean)
- Crumbled and cooked, turkey bacon, 6 slices, (1/2 lean)
- Cream cheese, low fat, 4 oz. (4 healthy fats)
- Diced canned jalapenos, 3 oz., (3 optional snacks)
- Garlic powder, 1/2 tsp. (1 condiment)
- Onion powder, 1/2 tsp. (1 condiment)
- Parmesan cheese, grated, 1/4 cup, (4 condiments)
- Sharp cheddar cheese, low fat, shredded and divided, 1 cup, (1 Lean)

Directions:

1. Heat the oven to 375 degrees.

2. Mix yogurt, shredded chicken, and cream cheese in a bowl.

3. Put in diced jalapenos, crumbled turkey bacon, onion powder, garlic powder, 1/2 cup cheddar cheese, and parmesan cheese.

4. Mix until fully blended. The mixture should be poured into a baking dish.

5. Adorn with the leftover 1/2 cup cheddar cheese.

6. Cook until cheese melts.

Nutrition:

Energy (calories): 12 kcal Protein: 0.78 g

Fat: 0.89 g Carbohydrates: 0.29 g

Taco Meatballs & Cheese Starters

Preparation Time:

10 minutes

Cooking Time:

30 minutes

Servings: 3

Ingredients:

- Ground beef, 95 to 97%, 16 oz. – cooks down to 12 oz., (2 leaner)
- Egg beaters, 1/4 cup
- Taco seasoning, 1 tbsp., (6 condiments)
- Cilantro, chopped, 1/4 cup
- Cheddar cheese in cubes, 5 oz., 2%, (7/8 Lean)
- For Dip:
- Sour cream, 1/4 cup (equals 2 Healthy Fats)
- Salsa, 2 tbsp. (equals 2 Condiments)

Directions:

1. Mix the egg beaters, ground beef, taco seasoning, and cilantro in a big bowl.
2. Make meatballs and put them onto a baking tray sprayed with nonstick.
3. Cook for about 15 minutes, at 425 degrees, till done. Set aside to cool.

4. Mix salsa and sour cream, put aside.
5. Equally divide the cheese cubes and meatballs into three portions.
6. Eat the portions with two tablespoons of salsa dip and sour cream.

Nutrition:

Energy (calories): 38 kcal Protein: 3.3 g

Fat: 1.47 g --Carbohydrates: 2.25 g

Avocado Chicken Salad

Preparation Time:

10 minutes

Cooking Time:

0 minutes

Servings: 2

Ingredients:

- Diced chicken, 10 oz., it's about 2 cups but for precision, weigh, (1 2/3 lean)
- Greek yogurt, plain, 1/2 cup 2% (1/3 lean)
- Chopped avocado, 3 oz., (2 healthy fats)
- Garlic powder, 1/2 tsp., (1 condiment)
- Salt, 1/4 tsp., (1 condiment)
- Pepper, 1/8 tsp., (1/2 condiment)
- Lime juice, 1 tbsp. + 1 tsp., (2 condiments)
- Chopped fresh cilantro, 1/4 cup (1/4 Condiment)

Directions:

1. In a medium-sized bowl, mix all the ingredients.
2. Put in the fridge till it's ready to be served.

3. Divide the chicken salad into halves and eat with greens of your choice!

Nutrition:

Energy (calories): 85 kcal Protein: 0.37 g

Fat: 0.66 g Carbohydrates: 0.38 g

Shrimp and Avocado Lettuce Wraps

Preparation Time:

15 minutes

Cooking Time:

6 minutes

Servings: 4

Ingredients:

- 2 pounds (907 g) raw shrimp, peeled and deveined
- 1 tablespoon Old Bay blackened seasoning
- 4 teaspoons olive oil, divided
- 6 ounces (170 g) avocado
- 1 cup plain Greek yogurt
- 2 tablespoons lime juice, divided
- 11/2 cups diced tomato
- 1/4 cup diced green bell pepper
- 1/4 cup chopped cilantro
- 1 jalapeño pepper, chopped and deseeded
- 1/4 cup chopped red onion
- 12 large romaine lettuce leaves

Directions:

1. Place shrimp and Old Bay seasoning in a resealable plastic bag. Shake to coat well.

2. Heat 2 teaspoons of olive oil in a skillet and add the shrimp.

3. Cook for 5 minutes on both sides or until shrimp are pink and cooked through.

4. You may need to work in batches to avoid overcrowding.

5. Combine the avocado, Greek yogurt, and 1 tablespoon of lime juice in a food processor. Pulse until smooth.

6. Stir the tomatoes, green bell pepper, cilantro, jalapeño pepper, onion, and remaining tablespoon of lime juice in a medium bowl.

7. Divide the shrimp, avocado mixture, and tomato mixture among the lettuce leaves.

8. Serve immediately.

Seared Scallops over Zucchini Noodles

Preparation Time:

10 minutes

Cooking Time:

15 minutes

Servings: 2

Ingredients:

- 2 small zucchinis, ends removed, and spiralized
- 1/2 tablespoon butter
- 1 pound (454 g) raw scallops
- 1/8 teaspoon salt
- Sauce:
- 6 ounces (170 g) jarred roasted red peppers, drained
- 2 ounces (57 g) avocado
- 1/2 cup unsweetened almond or cashew milk
- 2 teaspoons lemon juice
- 1 clove garlic
- 1/4 teaspoon salt
- 1/4 teaspoon crushed red pepper (optional)

Directions:

1. Combine all the sauce ingredients in a blender and purée until smooth.

2. Heat the roasted red pepper sauce in a skillet over medium heat, stirring occasionally, until heated through, about 3 to 5 minutes.

3. Stir in the zucchini noodles and continue to cook for an additional 3 to 5 minutes, or until cooked to your preference.

4. Meanwhile, melt the butter in a large skillet over medium-high heat.

5. Season the scallops with salt.

6. Cook the scallops until golden brown on each side and translucent in the center, about 1 to 2 minutes per side.

7. Serve the scallops over the zucchini noodles.

Nutrition: 1 Leanest 3 Greens 2 Healthy Fats 2 Condiments

Lemon Garlic Chicken Thighs with Asparagus

Preparation Time:

5 minutes

Cooking Time:

40 minutes

Servings: 4

Ingredients:

- 1¾ pounds (794 g) bone-in, skinless chicken thighs
- 2 tablespoons lemon juice
- 2 tablespoons minced fresh oregano
- 2 cloves garlic, minced
- 1/4 teaspoon pepper
- 1/4 teaspoon salt
- 2 pounds (907 g) asparagus, trimmed

Directions:

1. Preheat the oven to 350ºF (180ºC).
2. Toss all the ingredients except the asparagus in a mixing bowl until combined.
3. Roast the chicken thighs in the preheated oven for about 40 minutes, or until it reaches an internal temperature of 165ºF (74ºC).

4. When cooked, remove the chicken thighs from the oven and set aside to cool.

5. Meanwhile, steam the asparagus in the microwave to the desired doneness.

6. Serve the asparagus with roasted chicken thighs.

Nutrition: 1 Lean 3 Greens 2 Condiments

Mediterranean Pork Pita Sandwich

Preparation Time:

5 minutes

Cooking Time:

10 Minutes

Servings: 6

Ingredients:

- 2 teaspoons olive oil, plus 1 tablespoon
- 2 cups packed baby spinach leaves, finely chopped
- 4 ounces mushrooms, finely chopped
- 1 teaspoon chopped garlic
- 1 pound extra-lean ground pork
- 1 large egg
- ½ cup panko bread crumbs
- ⅓ cup chopped fresh dill
- ¼ teaspoon kosher salt
- 6 large romaine lettuce leaves, ripped into pieces to fit pita
- 2 tomatoes, sliced
- 3 whole-wheat pitas, cut in half
- ¾ cup Garlic Yogurt Sauce

Directions:

1. Heat 2 teaspoons of oil in a -inch skillet over medium heat.

2. Once the oil is shimmering, add the spinach, mushrooms, and garlic and sauté for 3 minutes. Cool for 5 minutes.

3. Place the mushroom mixture in a large mixing bowl and add the pork, egg, bread crumbs, dill, and salt.

4. Mix with your hands until everything is well combined. Make 6 patties, about ½-inch thick and 3 inches in diameter.

5. Heat the remaining 1 tablespoon of oil in the same 12-inch skillet over medium-high heat. When the oil is hot, add the patties.

6. They should all be able to fit in the pan. If not, cook in 2 batches. Cook for 5 minutes on the first side and 4 minutes on the second side. The outside should be golden brown, and the inside should no longer be pink.

7. Place 1 patty in each of 6 containers. In each of 6 separate containers that will not be reheated, place 1 torn lettuce leaf and 2 tomato slices.

8. Wrap the pita halves in plastic wrap and place one in each veggie container. Spoon 2 tablespoons of yogurt sauce into each of 6 sauce containers.

9. STORAGE: Store covered containers in the refrigerator for up to days. Uncooked patties can be frozen for up to 4 months, while cooked patties can be frozen for up to 3 months.

Nutrition Info: For Serving :
- Total calories: 309;
- Total fat: 11g;
- Saturated fat: 3g;
- Sodium: 343mg;
- Carbohydrates: 22g;
- Fiber: 3g;
- Protein: 32 g

Salmon With Warm Tomato-olive Salad

Preparation Time:

5 minutes

Cooking Time:

25 Minutes

Servings: 4

Ingredients:

- Salmon fillets (4/approx. 4 oz./1.25-inches thick)
- Celery (1 cup)
- Medium tomatoes (2)
- Fresh mint (.25 cup)
- Kalamata olives (.5 cup)
- Garlic (.5 tsp.)
- Salt (1 tsp. + more to taste)
- Honey (1 tbsp.)
- Red pepper flakes (.25 tsp.)
- Olive oil (2 tbsp. + more for the pan)
- Vinegar (1 tsp.)

Directions:

1. Slice the tomatoes and celery into inch pieces and mince the garlic. Chop the mint and the olives.

2. Heat the oven using the broiler setting.

3. Whisk the oil, vinegar, honey, red pepper flakes, and salt (1 tsp.. Brush the mixture onto the salmon.

4. Line the broiler pan with a sheet of foil. Spritz the pan lightly with olive oil, and add the fillets (skin side downward.

5. Broil them for four to six minutes until well done.

6. Meanwhile, make the tomato salad. Mix ½ teaspoon of the salt with the garlic.

7. Prepare a small saucepan on the stovetop using the med-high temperature setting. Pour in the rest of the oil and add the garlic mixture with the olives and one tablespoon of vinegar. Simmer for about three minutes.

8. Prepare the serving dishes. Pour the bubbly mixture into the bowl and add the mint, tomato, and celery. Dust it with the salt as desired and toss.

9. When the salmon is done, serve with a tomato salad.

Nutrition: Calories: 433; Protein: 38 grams; Fat: 26 grams

Mediterranean Minestrone Soup

Preparation Time:

10 minutes

Cooking Time:

40 Minutes

Servings: 4

Ingredients:

- 1 large onion, finely chopped
- 4 cups vegetable stock
- 4 cloves crushed garlic
- 1 ounce chopped carrots
- 4 ounces chopped red bell pepper
- 4 ounces chopped celery (keep leaves)
- 1 16-ounce can diced tomatoes
- 1 16-ounce can white beans
- 4 ounces fresh spinach, chopped
- 4 ounces multi-colored pasta
- 2 ounces grated parmesan
- 2 tablespoons olive oil
- bunch of chopped parsley
- 1 teaspoon dried oregano
- salt
- pepper
- 4 ounces salami, finely sliced (if desired)

Directions:

1. Heat oil in a pan over medium heat.
2. Add chopped onions, red pepper, carrots, and celery.
3. Saute for about 10 minutes until tender.
4. Add garlic and cook on low heat for 2 minutes more.
5. Add your stock and tomatoes and cook for an additional 10 minutes.
6. Add pasta and cook for 15 minutes more until al dente.
7. Taste / check your seasoning; add salt and pepper as needed.
8. Add parsley, beans, celery leaves, spinach, and salami (if using), and stir.
9. Pour the whole mixture to a boil and stir for about 2 minutes.
10. Enjoy the soup hot!

Nutrition: Calories: 888, Total Fat: 19.9 g, Saturated Fat: 6.3 g, Cholesterol: 30 mg, Sodium: 1200 mg, Total Carbohydrate: 139.5 g, Dietary Fiber: 31.8 g, Total Sugars: 14.3 g, Protein: 49.4 g, Vitamin D: 14 mcg, Calcium: 64.3 mg, Iron: 22 mg, Potassium: 3951 mg

Baked Shrimp Stew

Preparation Time:

5 minutes

Cooking Time:

25 Minutes

Servings: 4- 6

Ingredients:

- Greek extra virgin olive oil
- 2 1/2 lb prawns, peeled, deveined, rinsed well and dried
- 1 large red onion, chopped (about two cups)
- 5 garlic cloves, roughly chopped
- 1 red bell pepper, seeded, chopped
- 2 15-oz cans diced tomatoes
- 1/2 cup water
- 1 1/2 tsp ground coriander
- 1 tsp sumac
- 1 tsp cumin
- 1 tsp red pepper flakes, more to taste
- 1/2 tsp ground green cardamom
- Salt and pepper, to taste
- 1 cup parsley leaves, stems removed
- 1/3 cup toasted pine nuts
- 1/4 cup toasted sesame seeds

- Lemon or lime wedges to serve

Directions:

1. Preheat the oven to 375 degrees F
2. In a large frying pan, add 1 tbsp olive oil
3. Sauté the prawns for 2 minutes, until they are barely pink, then remove and set aside
4. In the same pan over medium-high heat, drizzle a little more olive oil and sauté the chopped onions, garlic and red bell peppers for 5 minutes, stirring regularly
5. Add in the canned diced tomatoes and water, allow to simmer for 10 minutes, until the liquid reduces, stir occasionally
6. Reduce the heat to medium, add the shrimp back to the pan, stir in the spices the ground coriander, sumac, cumin, red pepper flakes, green cardamom, salt and pepper, then the toasted pine nuts, sesame seeds and parsley leaves, stir to combined
7. Transfer the shrimp and sauce to an oven-safe earthenware or stoneware dish, cover tightly with foil Place in the oven to bake for minutes, uncover and broil briefly.
8. allow the dish to cool completely
9. Distribute among the containers, store for 2-3 days

10. To Serve: Reheat on the stove for 1-2 minutes or until heated through. Serve with your favorite bread or whole grain. Garnish with a side of lime or lemon wedges.

Nutrition: Calories:377;Carbs: ;Total Fat: 20g;Protein: 41g

Rainbow Salad With Roasted Chickpeas

Preparation Time:

5 minutes

Cooking Time:

40 Minutes

Servings: 2 - 3

Ingredients:

- Creamy avocado dressing, store bought or homemade
- 3 large tri-color carrots - one orange, one red, and one yellow
- 1 medium zucchini
- 1/4 cup fresh basil, cut into ribbons
- 1 can chickpeas, rinsed and drained
- 1 tbsp olive oil
- 1 tsp chili powder
- 1/2 tsp cumin
- Salt, to taste
- Pepper, to taste

Directions:

1. Preheat the oven to 400 degrees F
2. Pat the chickpeas dry with paper towels

3. Add them to a bowl and toss with the olive oil, chili powder, cumin, and salt and pepper

4. Arrange the chickpeas on a baking sheet in a single layer

5. Bake for 30-40 minutes - making sure to shaking the pan once in a while to prevent over browning. The chickpeas will be done when they're crispy and golden brown, allow to cool

6. With a grater, peeler, mandolin or spiralizer, shred the carrots and zucchini into very thin ribbons

7. Once the zucchini is shredded, lightly press it with paper towels to remove excess moisture

8. Add the shredded zucchini and carrots to a bowl, toss with the basil

9. Add in the roasted chickpeas, too gently to combine

10. Distribute among the containers.

11. To Serve: Top with the avocado dress

Nutrition Calories: 640; Total Fat: 51g; Total Carbs: 9.8g; Protein: 38.8g

Sour And Sweet Fish

Preparation Time:

5 minutes

Cooking Time:

25 Minutes

Servings: 2

Ingredients:

- 1 tablespoon vinegar
- 2 drops stevia
- 1 pound fish chunks
- ¼ cup butter, melted
- Salt and black pepper, to taste

Directions:

1. Put butter and fish chunks in a skillet and cook for about 3 minutes.
2. Add stevia, salt and black pepper and cook for about 10 minutes, stirring continuously.
3. Dish out in a bowl and serve immediately.
4. Place fish in a dish and set aside to cool for meal prepping.
5. Divide it in 2 containers and refrigerate for up to 2 days.
6. Reheat in microwave before serving.

Nutrition: Calories: 2; Carbohydrates: 2.8g; Protein: 24.5g; Fat: 16.7g; Sugar: 2.7g; Sodium: 649mg

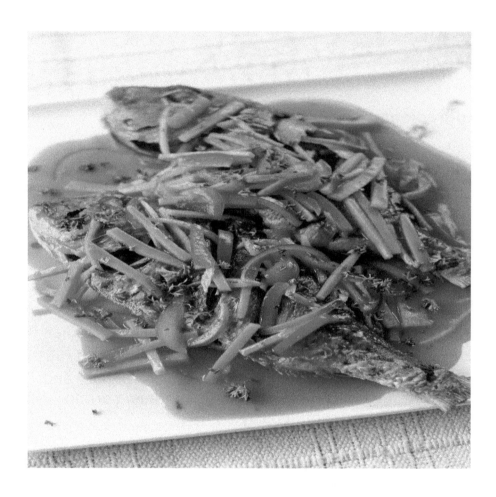

Papaya Mangetout Stew

Preparation Time:

5 minutes

Cooking Time:

5 Minutes

Servings: 2

Ingredients:

- 2 cups Mangetout
- 2 cups bean sprouts
- 1 tablespoon water
- 1 papaya, peeled, deseeded, and cubed
- 1 lime, juiced
- 2 tablespoon unsalted peanuts
- small handful basil leaves, torn
- small handful mint leaves, chopped

Directions:

1. Take a large frying pan and place it over high heat.
2. Add Mangetout, 1 tablespoon of water, and bean sprouts.
3. Cook for about 2-minutes.
4. Remove from heat, add papaya, and lime juice.
5. Toss everything well.
6. Spread over containers.

7. Before eating, garnish with herbs and peanuts.
8. Enjoy!

Nutrition: Calories: 283, Total Fat: 6.4 g, Saturated Fat: 0.g, Cholesterol: 0 mg, Sodium: 148 mg, Total Carbohydrate: 42.8 g, Dietary Fiber: 4.9 g, Total Sugars: 21.5 g, Protein: 20.1 g, Vitamin D: 0 mcg, Calcium: 205 mg, Iron: 3 mg, Potassium: 743 mg

Tilapia with Smoked Gouda

Preparation Time:

5 minutes

Cooking Time:

40 minutes

Servings: 6

Ingredients:

- 1 shallot
- 1 cup fish stock
- 2 turnips
- 1 leek
- 3 cloves garlic
- 1 1/4 pound tilapia
- 6 medium-sized tomatoes
- 1/4 bunch parsley
- 1/4 cup red wine
- 1 teaspoon olive oil
- 3 ounces of smoked Gouda

Directions:

1. Wash and rinse the fish in ice water.
2. Dice all the tomatoes; remove the covering of the turnips.
3. Slice leek, mince all the shallot and the garlic, make the parsley chopped, and the cheese should be grated

4. Put olive oil inside the baking dish, place shallot, garlic, fish, and turnip. Add the wine and stock, also bake for 30 minutes

5. Open the cover and add cheese and tomatoes.

6. Put it back inside the oven until the cheese has melted. It is ready to be served.

Nutrition:

- Calories: 100
- Carbs: 52 g
- Fat: 2 g
- Protein: 20 g

Cauliflower Soup with Seeds

Preparation Time:

10 minutes

Cooking Time:

20 minutes

Servings: 4

Ingredients:

- 2 cups cauliflower
- 1 tablespoon pumpkin seeds
- 1 tablespoon chia seeds
- 1/2 teaspoon salt
- 1 teaspoon butter
- 1/4 white onion, diced
- 1/2 cup coconut cream
- 1 cup of water
- 4 ounces Parmesan, grated
- 1 teaspoon paprika
- 1 tablespoon dried cilantro

Directions:

1. Chop cauliflower and put it in the saucepan.
2. Add salt, butter, diced onion, paprika, and dried cilantro.

3. Cook the cauliflower over medium heat for 5 minutes.

4. Then add coconut cream and water.

5. Close the lid and boil soup for 15 minutes.

6. Then blend the soup with the help of a hand blender.

7. Ding to boil it again.

8. Add grated cheese and mix up well.

9. Spoon the soup and top every bowl with pumpkin seeds and chia seeds.

Nutrition:

- Calories: 214
- Fat: 16.4 g
- Fiber: 3.6 g
- Carbs: 8.1 g
- Protein: 12.1 g

Prosciutto-Wrapped Asparagus

Preparation Time:

15 minutes

Cooking Time:

20 minutes

Servings: 6

Ingredients:

- 2-pound asparagus
- 8 ounces prosciutto, sliced
- 1 tablespoon butter, melted
- 1/2 teaspoon ground black pepper
- 4 tablespoon heavy cream
- 1 tablespoon lemon juice

Directions:

1. Slice prosciutto slices into strips.
2. Wrap asparagus into prosciutto strips and place them on the tray.
3. Sprinkle the vegetables with ground black pepper, heavy cream, and lemon juice. Add butter.
4. Preheat the oven to 365°F.
5. Place the tray with asparagus in the oven and cook for 20 minutes.
6. Serve the cooked meal only hot.

Nutrition:

- Calories: 138
- Fat: 7.9 g
- Fiber: 3.2 g
- Carbs: 6.9 g
- Protein: 11.5 g

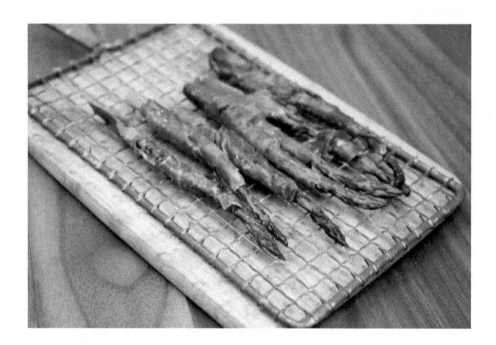

Stuffed Bell Peppers

Preparation Time:

10 minutes

Cooking Time:

25 minutes

Servings: 4

Ingredients:

- 4 bell peppers
- 1 1/2 cup ground beef
- 1 zucchini, grated
- 1 white onion, diced
- 1/2 teaspoon ground nutmeg
- 1 tablespoon olive oil
- 1 teaspoon ground black pepper
- 1/2 teaspoon salt
- 3 ounces Parmesan, grated

Directions:

1. Slit the peppers into halves and remove the seeds.
2. Place the ground beef in the skillet.
3. Add grated zucchini, diced onion, ground nutmeg, olive oil, ground black pepper, and salt.
4. Roast the mixture for 5 minutes.

5. Place bell pepper halves in the tray.

6. Fill every pepper half with ground beef mixture and top with grated Parmesan.

7. Cover the tray with foil and secure the edges.

8. Cook the stuffed bell peppers for 20 minutes at 360°F.

Nutrition:

- Calories: 241
- Fat: 14.6 g
- Fiber: 3.4 g
- Carbs: 11 g
- Protein: 18.6 g

Stuffed Eggplants with Goat Cheese

Preparation Time:

15 minutes

Cooking Time:

25 minutes

Servings: 4

Ingredients:

- 1 large eggplant, trimmed
- 1 tomato, crushed
- 1 garlic clove, diced
- 1/2 teaspoon ground black pepper
- 1/2 teaspoon smoked paprika
- 1 cup spinach, chopped
- 4 ounces goat cheese, crumbled
- 1 teaspoon butter
- 2 ounces cheddar cheese, shredded

Directions:

1. Cut the eggplants into halves and then cut every half into 2 parts.
2. Remove the flesh from the eggplants to get eggplant boards.
3. Mix up together crushed tomato, diced garlic, ground black pepper, smoked paprika, chopped spinach, crumbled goat cheese, and butter.

4. Fill the eggplants with this mixture.

5. Top every eggplant board with shredded cheddar cheese.

6. Put the eggplants in the tray.

7. Preheat the oven to 365°F.

8. Place the tray with eggplants in the oven and cook for 25 minutes.

Nutrition:

- Calories: 229
- Fat: 16 g
- Fiber: 4.6 g
- Carbs: 9 g
- Protein: 13.8 g

Korma Curry

Preparation Time:

10 minutes

Cooking Time:

25 minutes

Servings: 6

Ingredients:

- 3-pound chicken breast, skinless, boneless
- 1 teaspoon gram masala
- 1 teaspoon curry powder
- 1 tablespoon apple cider vinegar
- 1/2 coconut cream
- 1 cup organic almond milk
- 1 teaspoon ground coriander
- 3/4 teaspoon ground cardamom
- 1/2 teaspoon ginger powder
- 1/4 teaspoon cayenne pepper
- 3/4 teaspoon ground cinnamon
- 1 tomato, diced
- 1 teaspoon avocado oil
- 1/2 cup of water

Directions:

1. Chop the chicken breast and put it in the saucepan.

2. Add avocado oil and start to cook it over medium heat.

3. Sprinkle the chicken with gram masala, curry powder, apple cider vinegar, ground coriander, cardamom, ginger powder, cayenne pepper, ground cinnamon, and diced tomato.

4. Mix up the ingredients carefully. Cook them for 10 minutes.

5. Add water, coconut cream, and almond milk. Sauté the meal for 10 minutes more.

Nutrition:

- Calories: 411
- Fat: 19.3 g
- Fiber: 0.9 g
- Carbs: 6 g
- Protein: 49.9 g

Zucchini Bars

Preparation Time:

10 minutes

Cooking Time:

15 minutes

Servings: 8

Ingredients:

- 3 zucchini, grated
- 1/2 white onion, diced
- 2 teaspoons butter
- 3 eggs, whisked
- 4 tablespoons coconut flour
- 1 teaspoon salt
- 1/2 teaspoon ground black pepper
- 5 ounces goat cheese, crumbled
- 4 ounces Swiss cheese, shredded
- 1/2 cup spinach, chopped
- 1 teaspoon baking powder
- 1/2 teaspoon lemon juice

Directions:

1. In the mixing bowl, mix up together grated zucchini, diced onion, eggs, coconut flour, salt, ground black pepper, crumbled cheese, chopped

spinach, baking powder, and lemon juice.

2. Add butter and churn the mixture until homogenous.
3. Line the baking dish with baking paper.
4. Transfer the zucchini mixture into the baking dish and flatten it.
5. Preheat the oven to 365°F and put the dish inside.
6. Cook it for 15 minutes. Then chill the meal well.
7. Cut it into bars.

Nutrition:

- Calories: 199
- Fat: 1316 g
- Fiber: 215 g
- Carbs: 7.1 g
- Protein: 13.1 g

Mushroom Soup

Preparation Time:

10 minutes

Cooking Time:

25 minutes

Servings: 4

Ingredients:

- 1 cup water
- 1 cup coconut milk
- 1 cup white mushrooms, chopped
- 1/2 carrot, chopped
- 1/4 white onion, diced
- 1 tablespoon butter
- 2 ounces turnip, chopped
- 1 teaspoon dried dill
- 1/2 teaspoon ground black pepper
- 3/4 teaspoon smoked paprika
- 1 ounce celery stalk, chopped

Directions:

1. Pour water and coconut milk into the saucepan. Bring the liquid to a boil.
2. Add chopped mushrooms, carrots, and turnip. Boil for 10 minutes.

3. Meanwhile, put butter in the skillet. Add diced onion.
4. Sprinkle it with dill, ground black pepper, and smoked paprika.
5. Roast the onion for 3 minutes.
6. Add the roasted onion to the soup mixture.
7. Then add chopped celery stalk. Close the lid.
8. Cook soup for 10 minutes.
9. Then ladle it into the serving bowls.

Nutrition:

- Calories: 181
- Fat: 17.3 g
- Fiber: 2.5 g
- Carbs: 6.9 g
- Protein: 2.4 g

Stuffed Portobello Mushrooms

Preparation Time:

10 minutes

Cooking Time:

10 minutes

Servings: 4

Ingredients:

- 2 Portobello mushrooms
- 1 cup spinach, chopped, steamed
- 2 ounces artichoke hearts, drained, chopped
- 1 tablespoon coconut cream
- 1 tablespoon cream cheese
- 1 teaspoon minced garlic
- 1 tablespoon fresh cilantro, chopped
- 3 ounces Cheddar cheese, grated
- 1/2 teaspoon ground black pepper
- 2 tablespoons olive oil
- 1/2 teaspoon salt

Directions:

1. Sprinkle mushrooms with olive oil and place them in the tray.

2. Transfer the tray in the preheated to 360°F oven and broil them for 5 minutes.

3. Meanwhile, blend together artichoke hearts, coconut cream, cream cheese, minced garlic, and chopped cilantro.

4. Add grated cheese in the mixture and sprinkle with ground black pepper and salt.

5. Fill the broiled mushrooms with the cheese mixture and cook them for 5 minutes more.

6. Serve the mushrooms only hot.

Nutrition:

- Calories: 183
- Fat: 16.3 g
- Fiber: 1.9 g
- Carbs: 3 g
- Protein: 7.7 g

Lettuce Salad

Preparation Time:

10 minutes

Cooking Time:

10 minutes

Servings: 1

Ingredients:

- 1 cup Romaine lettuce, roughly chopped
- 3 ounces seitan, chopped
- 1 tablespoon avocado oil
- 1 teaspoon sunflower seeds
- 1 teaspoon lemon juice
- 1 egg, boiled, peeled
- 2 ounces cheddar cheese, shredded

Directions:

1. Place lettuce in the salad bowl.
2. Add chopped seitan and shredded cheese.
3. Then chop the egg roughly and add to the salad bowl too.
4. Mix up together lemon juice with the avocado oil.

5. Sprinkle the salad with the oil mixture and sunflower seeds.

6. Don't stir the salad before serving.

Nutrition:

- Calories: 663
- Fat: 29.5 g
- Fiber: 4.7 g
- Carbs: 3.8 g
- Protein: 84.2 g

Onion Soup

Preparation Time:

10 minutes

Cooking Time:

25 minutes

Servings: 6

Ingredients:

- 2 cups white onion, diced
- 4 tablespoon butter
- 1/2 cup white mushrooms, chopped
- 3 cups water
- 1 cup heavy cream
- 1 teaspoon salt
- 1 teaspoon chili flakes
- 1 teaspoon garlic powder

Directions:

1. Put butter in the saucepan and melt it.
2. Add diced white onion, chili flakes, and garlic powder.
3. Mix it up and sauté for 10 minutes over medium-low heat.
4. Then add water, heavy cream, and chopped mushrooms. Close the lid.
5. Cook the soup for 15 minutes more.

6. Then blend the soup until you get the creamy texture. Ladle it in the bowls.

Nutrition:

- Calories: 155
- Fat: 15.1 g
- Fiber: 0.9 g
- Carbs: 4.7 g

  Protein: 1.2 g

Asparagus Salad

Preparation Time:

10 minutes

Cooking Time:

15 minutes

Servings: 3

Ingredients:

- 10 ounces asparagus
- 1 tablespoon olive oil
- 1/2 teaspoon white pepper
- 4 ounces feta cheese, crumbled
- 1 cup lettuce, chopped
- 1 tablespoon canola oil
- 1 teaspoon apple cider vinegar
- 1 tomato, diced

Directions:

1. Preheat the oven to 365°F.
2. Place asparagus in the tray, sprinkle with olive oil and white pepper and transfer it to the preheated oven.
3. Cook it for 15 minutes.
4. Meanwhile, put crumbled feta in the salad bowl.
5. Add chopped lettuce and diced tomato.

6. Sprinkle the ingredients with apple cider vinegar.

7. Chill the cooked asparagus to room temperature and add in the salad.

8. Shake the salad gently before serving.

Nutrition:

- Calories: 207
- Fat: 17.6 g
- Fiber: 2.4 g
- Carbs: 6.8 g
- Protein: 7.8 g

Cauliflower Tabbouleh

Preparation Time:

10 minutes

Cooking Time:

4 minutes

Servings: 4

Ingredients:

- 1-pound cauliflower head
- 1 cucumber, chopped
- 2 tablespoons lemon juice
- 2 tablespoons olive oil
- 1/2 cup fresh parsley
- 1 garlic clove, diced
- 1 ounce scallions, chopped
- 1 teaspoon mint

Directions:

1. Trim and chop cauliflower head. Transfer it to the food processor and pulse until you get cauliflower rice.
2. Transfer the cauliflower rice to the glass mixing bowl.
3. Add lemon juice and chopped scallions. Mix up the mixture.
4. Microwave it for 4 minutes.

5. Meanwhile, blend together olive oil, parsley, and diced garlic.

6. Mix up together cooked cauliflower rice with parsley mixture.

7. Add mint and chopped cucumbers.

8. Mix it up and transfer it to the serving plates.

Nutrition:

- Calories: 108
- Fat: 7.3 g
- Fiber: 3.7 g
- Carbs: 10.2 g
- Protein: 3.2 g

Stuffed Artichoke

Preparation Time:

10 minutes

Cooking Time:

15 minutes

Servings: 4

Ingredients:

- 2 artichokes
- 4 tablespoon Parmesan, grated
- 2 teaspoon almond flour
- 1 teaspoon minced garlic
- 3 tablespoons sour cream
- 1 teaspoon avocado oil
- 1 cup water, for cooking

Directions:

1. Set water in the saucepan and let it boil.
2. When the water is boiling, add artichokes and boil them for 5 minutes.
3. Drain water from artichokes and trim them.
4. Remove the artichoke hearts.
5. Preheat the oven to 365°F.

6. Mix up together almond flour, grated Parmesan, minced garlic, sour cream, and avocado oil.

7. Fill the artichokes with cheese mixture and place them on the baking tray.

8. Cook the vegetables for 10 minutes.

9. Then cut every artichoke into halves and transfer it to the serving plates.

Nutrition:

- Calories: 162
- Fat: 10.7 g
- Fiber: 5.9 g
- Carbs: 12.4 g
- Protein: 8.2 g

Beef Salpicao

Preparation Time:

10 minutes

Cooking Time:

18 minutes

Servings: 2

Ingredients:

- 1-pound rib eye, boneless
- 2 garlic cloves, peeled, diced
- 2 tablespoons butter
- 1 tablespoon sour cream
- 1/2 teaspoon salt
- 1/2 teaspoon chili pepper
- 1 tablespoon lime juice

Directions:

1. Cut rib eye into the strips.
2. Sprinkle the meat with salt, chili pepper, and lime juice.
3. Toss butter in the skillet.
4. Add diced garlic and roast it for 2 minutes over medium heat.
5. Then add meat strips and roast them over high heat for 2 minutes from each side.

6. Add sour cream and close the lid.
7. Cook the meal for 10 minutes more over medium heat.
8. Stir it from time to time.
9. Transfer the cooked beef Salpicao to the serving plates.

Nutrition:

- Calories: 641
- Fat: 52.8 g
- Fiber: 0.1 g
- Carbs: 1.9 g
- Protein: 42.5 g

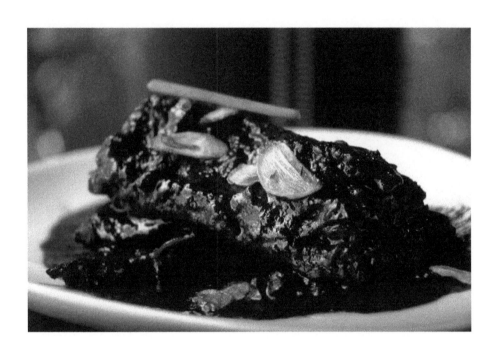